Detoxing With Cannabis

Easy Natural Weight Loss

My 10 year adventure to find a
true detox weight loss CURE that I
could do in the comfort of my own home.

In Five Chapters.

Detoxing With Cannabis by Don Endriss

Copyright 2017

DonsSuperFlush.com

Contents

This book is written for people who legally use low THC Sativa strands of medical grade Cannabis to supplement their health.

If you're a medical marijuana patient who wants to lose weight while also flushing out old water soluble toxins, then this book is for you.

I'm not interested in getting high. I want reliably produced low THC medical grade cannabis for detoxing purposes only!

I hope you're able to attain the same level of success with your health that I've achieved.

Everyone else should consider this book to be pure science fiction entertainment, literary art.

Either way, turn the page and prepare to smile ☺

I won't let you down!

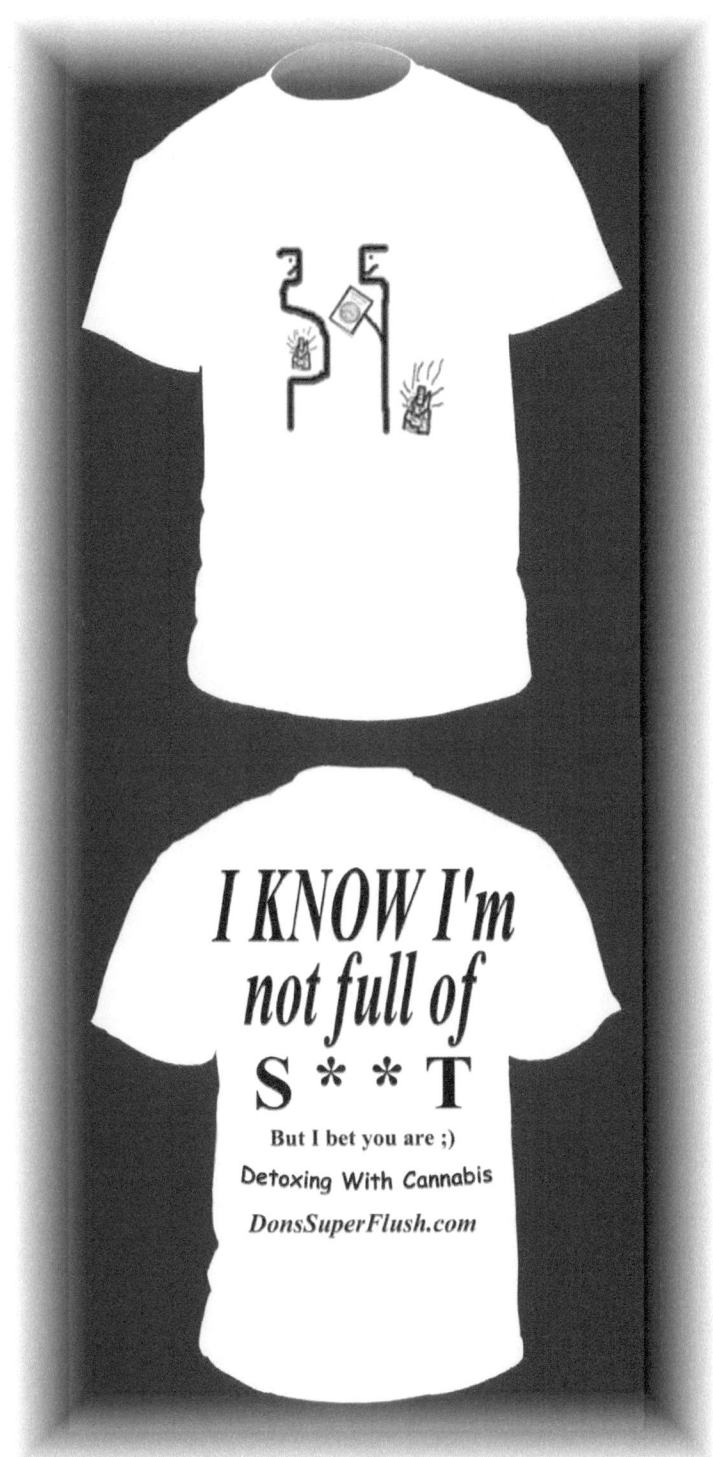

1 - Detoxing With Cannabis

How I slowly lost 100 pounds, quit smoking, and got back into shape.

The purpose of this book is not to serve as a therapeutic guide. I am not a doctor nor do I have any medical training. You should consult with your physician before trying anything you read here, especially if you're currently under the care of a physician.

I am simply a student of life trying to improve my health as my body grows older. It's time to start a new discussion on removing toxic waste from our system. My thoughts are merely observations and not expert explanations.

I wish I could have found a detox book like this in the beginning of my journey. I would have liked some simple guidance on how to cleanse out years of toxic build up from within my system. Read this book or follow my path at your own risk.

Agree or disagree with my Indicators, concepts and evidence. I quit smoking cigarettes, lost 100 pounds and kept it off for over two years while getting back into good physical shape. I believe IF the principles of cleansing and detoxifying with Sativa strands of medical-grade Cannabis were aired on main stream television, we would have a stronger, healthier and happier society in 3-5 years.

People say you are what you eat; I say maybe for those who lived a thousand years ago. But with today's processed foods your body is forced to contend with stabilizers, neutralizers, additives, and preservatives. Imagine eating a whole bowl of that stuff.

Year after year we gradually expose our bodies to more and more of these man-made toxins. Sprinkle by sprinkle they slowly add up to become a full bowl of chemicals. This is slow death for some of us. I say in today's world of chemically formulated fast foods, you actually become what your body is unable to get rid of.

Yet go into any grocery store and you'll find dozens of items for washing, repairing, brushing, cleaning, and flossing your mouth. All the stuff you need to keep the entrance looking clean and working nicely.

Sooner or later everything breaks down. Someday every cell in your body will need to be repaired or replaced. Whenever your body is fighting degradation or disease, there's always debris heading towards a trash can. When you become ill, chances are you're having trouble eliminating your waste. Fix the problem of backed up trash, and your body will have more energy to put towards fighting disease.

I believe most pain is caused from the bodies' inability to effectively remove its waste. If the body can't get rid of its waste, then that micro-force builds up. One day you'll start feeling the pressure. Sometimes I've had lower back pain disappear simply by doing a coffee cleanse. By getting rid of waste I also get rid of the pain.

Do you ever think about that old fat you put on years ago? It's still right there, as toxic as the day you made it. From what I've researched, the body doesn't trade old fat for new fat. No switch is made.

It's my belief that when the body builds these long standing fat cells, it uses whatever moisture is currently in your system. To me that says if water soluble toxins are in the moisture, then those toxins are getting blended into the fat cell mix.

This concept also applies to newly formed muscle. The only way I can think of to remove toxins from muscle is with hydration, dilation, exercise, stretching and elimination.

It's not just about the bad toxins you've eaten, there's also the self-made stress and rage toxins. Negative thoughts create toxins. These stress and rage toxins congeal and get mixed in with your newly formed muscle and fat.

I believe if you're in a stressful situation while creating these fat cells, then some of the water soluble stress toxins floating around your body can also become intertwined with your newly made fat cells. Building new fat cells gives these toxins a place to hide.

So years later when you're exercising and burning off that old fat, it releases those stored stress toxins. The alarm system goes off as the body recognizes the stress markers and your subconscious mind suddenly begins to relive old stress from years ago. Have you ever been angry or felt on edge while trying to lose weight?

The body does as it's told. You become the thoughts you think about all day. When old toxins and stress markers are suddenly reintroduced to the body through exercise and weight loss, your system prepares for some kind of battle. So you lose the weight but you find yourself in a constant state of emotional struggle.

If you are upset while eating that tub of ice cream, chances are you'll be a little upset when you burn those fat cells off. When it comes to weight loss, I believe the release of stress toxins is what most people struggle with.

If there's one pound of toxins spread throughout the body of a 400 lb person, and they lose 200 lbs without cleansing those toxins out, you now have one pound of toxins in a 200 lb person.

They'll be slimmer and trimmer but twice as physically and mentally toxic as they were before. Having a higher ratio of toxins in your system's chemistry makes you more susceptible to toxin-related diseases and mood disorders such as PTSD.

You think you're losing weight and getting skinny but your toxin levels rise with each pound lost. When you lose weight, you need to have a working plan for eliminating those old water soluble toxins being re-released.

If you don't, there's a strong chance they'll go right back into your system. Getting rid of water soluble toxins is EVERYONES' big problem and it's because of the way our lower colon functions.

I've read that when you detox, it can take the body up to ten times to remove water soluble toxins from your bile waste. That's ten times when you're TRYING to do it correctly and there's a reason why EVERYONE struggles!

"It's a physiological fact that bile is normally reabsorbed up to ten times by the body before working its way out of the intestine in feces." (Note #1) Dr. Max Gerson, Healing The Hopeless

It seems the lower intestine collects water and anything else the body can use just before elimination. So if you're dehydrated, those water soluble toxins get pulled right back into the distribution system.

Did you forget to drink some water before your workout and now you feel super dehydrated? Don't worry, your body will grab some moisture from that dirty toxic waste by the exit. Round and round it goes, and when it stops, only your actions will show. It explains why sometimes you feel angry or on edge while losing weight.

When your body is thirsty or hungry, it digs deep through whatever is in the pipeline. Many of those water soluble toxins are re-absorbed from the body's attempt to retrieve and recycle every last drop of water and nutrition. So if you starve yourself and you only drink water after your workouts and not during them, chances are you're miserable and I bet it's because of toxins.

Imagine your body working to kick those toxins out. Then during exercise, those toxins come floating right back in because you're dehydrated. Your body is constantly fighting a losing battle during the elimination process.

Those same toxins are being re-absorbed at the very last step, right before the exit.

That's why I like to do this detox cleanse regiment. It helps the toxic waste being released from exercise to bypass the function of the lower colon. It helps the lower colon by preventing it from grabbing any extra moisture loaded with these water soluble toxins.

A coffee cleanse allows everything that's sluggishly trapped behind the bile duct to swiftly pass through in one elimination flush. As I researched coffee cleanses I learned about Dr Max Gerson and his cancer fighting therapy.

"On arriving at the liver, the caffeine stimulated the opening of the bile ducts to increase the flow of bile, which removes toxins from the liver and deposits them into the small intestine, for eventual elimination in the feces. The unburdened liver is then free to remove more toxins from the bloodstream – one of the organ's most crucial normal functions." Charlotte Gerson and Morton Walker, The Gerson Therapy (Note #2)

I want everyone reading my book to understand that how I use elements of The Gerson coffee cleanse with Cannabis is not supported by the Gerson Institute. Using Cannabis for cleansing is my theory, and not a part of any other program that I am aware of.

I was drawn to the Gerson Therapy because of the miracle like results his case studies showed for curing cancer. My impression of "The Gerson Therapy" was that the less energy your body spends on getting rid of waste, the more energy it has to heal itself. That by drinking organic pressed juices, you are giving your body all the nutritional value of the plant, without taxing your energy supply to process the pulp.

Max Gerson studied and worked on the removal of waste from the lower colon with the use of coffee colon cleanses. When coffee is boiled, the grinds release their palmatic acid and oil that can dilate the opening of the bile duct, and along with glutathione S-transferase the body is able to increase toxin removal by up to 700%.

"Wattenberg and coworkers were able to prove in 1981 that the palmatic acid found in coffee promotes the activity of glutathione S-transferase and other ligands by manyfold times above the normal. It is this enzyme group which is responsible primarily for the conjugation of free electrophile radicals which the gall bladder will then release" Charlotte Gerson and Morton Walker, The Gerson Therapy (Note #3)

When the coffee oil stimulates the bile duct to open wide, it allows everything in there that's backed up to become saturated.

"This detoxifying of cancer cells has been demonstrated innumerable times by experiments on laboratory mice wherein detoxification of the liver increases by 600 percent and the small bowel detoxifies by 700 percent when coffee beans are added to the animals' diet. Analogous results take place within humans who are giving themselves coffee enemas." Charlotte Gerson and Morton Walker, The Gerson Therapy (Note #4)

I believe the sudden force of this sludge rushing away creates a small vacuum that tugs the future waste in the pipeline progressively closer towards the elimination path. That the coffee cleanse allows the system to give one big push, and that inertia generated suction potentially pulls on clogged and damaged pathways.

I thought, if this works for people who already have cancer, then perhaps there are some things I should incorporate into my daily schedule. Maybe I could better my odds for a healthier cancer-free life if I made some small changes in my daily routine. Since meeting that crossroad, I lost over 100 pounds and am able to exercise 5 days a week.

My thoughts began to revolve around three things. Fresh organic juices for work-free nutrition, dilation for moisture infusion and deep cell cleansing, and a coffee colon flush to get it all out. The routine I developed is a compilation of many different ideas and theories. All of the home therapies I do are well known.

I just figured out the tiny details of each step and tested their combinations to achieve maximum detox benefit for my body. It helps to understand HOW these three things Hydrate, Dilate and Eliminate work together to create a perfect cleansing storm, or should I say, (Drum Roll Please) – Don's Super Flush! Cleanse away your past stress toxins and close that door forever.

When I detox with medical-grade Sativa Cannabis, a process of removing backed up waste in my system begins. From start to finish it takes me about 3 hours to complete the evening portion of my micro-cleanse, and 90 minutes for the morning. So have patience with yourself. You'll be doing this twice, once in the evening and then again in the morning.

Pick a day of the week where you'll have some uninterrupted time to yourself. Three to four hours for the evening portion should give you plenty of time. Don't put on your white tuxedo and head for the dance floor after you finish. It's best to stay home and rest.

I like to do this on a Friday night and Saturday morning. The Friday night portion gets everything nice and loose for the AM. While you're sleeping, the body continues to move waste, and your Saturday morning Elimination gets the Friday night cell wash out.

I make a shopping list and get everything ready in the house before Friday, or what ever day you choose. Plan to have a healthy breakfast, lunch and dinner. It might take you all week to get set up, and that's OK, just get there. Maybe eat your favorite healthy dessert while watching your favorite funny movie! Well that's the basic overview of how to detox with Cannabis.

In the next chapters I reveal my tested plan for how each portion of this regiment is prepared. Learn from my mistakes. Once you understand what to look out for this entire process becomes very easy to do! Hydrate, Dilate, Eliminate, these three things done properly have become my miracle cure combination!

Open the door to good health and take the first step by reading my story. For the price of a healthy lunch, I share with you my ten year adventure to find a true weight loss toxin removal solution. Something that really works! Something you can do by yourself in the privacy of your own home.

I say start living as if there IS going to be a tomorrow. You'll be lighter, healthier and a heck of a lot happier! Cleanse your body and heal your mind. Detoxing With Cannabis, the do it yourself miracle home therapy that already saved a life, mine!

See how nature intended for you to look.

Notes

(Note #1) ~ From page 15 - Charlotte Gerson and Morton Walker, The Gerson Therapy, Kensington Books copyright 2001   Page 162   ISBN: 1-57566-628-6

(Note #2) ~ From page 16 - Dr. Max Gerson, Healing The Hopeless, Howard Straus with Barbara Marinacci, Kensington Books copyright 2001   Page 182   ISBN: 0976018616

(Note #3) ~   From page 17 - Charlotte Gerson and Morton Walker, The Gerson Therapy, Kensington Books copyright 2001   Page 160   ISBN: 1-57566-628-6

(Note #4) ~   From page 17 - Charlotte Gerson and Morton Walker, The Gerson Therapy, Kensington Books copyright 2001   Page 160   ISBN: 1-57566-628-6

I would like to say that I see the Gerson family and all the work they've done for mankind, as proof that angels do exist on earth. God bless the Gerson family and all those who help to spread Max Gerson's therapy.

2 – Hydrate

For us, there is no life without water!!!

As you read along from this point forward, I hope you won't judge me until I've finished making my case. Because in all my craziness, some how I'll find a way to make some interesting points. It's time to dive in; it's time to get started.

For the next three chapters I'll go into greater detail for each of the three major things you need to think about, Hydrating, Dilating, and Eliminating. And there's only one place to start, and that's with WATER! The first step is to hydrate. It's time to get the body filled with water, and it's important to make sure you do this correctly.

So when I'm positive that I have about 3-4 hours to myself with no interruptions, only then do I start hydrating by slowly drinking a 12 ounce glass of water every 20 minutes. Don't try to drink a lot of water very fast; SLOW and steady is the only way to get this job done right.

Do not over drink water or juice. You should be OK by the 3rd glass if you're of average build and 4th if you're big. The goal is to get enough water into your body so that the lower intestine does not absorb any of the coffee cleanse. I drink a lot of water and tea during the day, so most of the time I'm already hydrated.

Around my third glass I begin to feel full. At this point I believe my body has taken in enough water to reach a kind of equilibrium. Just FYI, at best most people can process 36 ounces of clean water in an hour. I drink one glass of juice and then the rest is water, not juice for all 3-4 glasses! I love fresh juice, but it's mostly about drinking clean water!

Remember that time when you took a sip of something so healthy and delicious that you actually felt energy transferring from your drink into your body? Well why not have a fresh organic juice, coconut water, a nice herbal tea, something like chamomile tea, and then switch over to water during that first hour.

Maybe have a fresh salad, your favorite fruit, or whatever is delicious and healthy to you. Have something that makes your body say wow! But if all you have is water, then you're in luck because water works great all by itself!

I use filtered tap water for making everything around the house, whether it's for cooking, drinking, or teas. I like green tea for the morning and then Chamomile tea for the evening. I am also a big fan of Earl Gray tea. It has an amazing list of health benefits, and I like to drink that when I do a 5-day juice fast. But my go-to tea is green tea, that gets me through the day with focus and drive.

If you're considering drinking juice, it should be freshly made from something that's connected to the earth, a tree, bush or plant. Something that carries life energy from the earth to its fruit. There's not much fresh life energy in a juice with a 45-day shelf life. Ever seen month old grapes, no one eats rotten old grapes, why would you drink them?

The best book on juicing that I've read so far is called "The Complete Book Of Juicing" by Michael T Murray, N.D. In chapter 8 he reminds us that,

"Hippocrates's, the father of western medicine, said, "Let your food be your medicine and let you medicine be your food." "It is amazing how far we have drifted from this sound advice". The Complete Book Of Juicing, Michael T. Murray, N.D. FORWORD By Jay Kordich, "The Juiceman". (Note #5)

Think about the earth's natural force coming up through the root into every piece of fruit. This energy cannot be duplicated with factory made processed sugar drinks. Consume something alive that carries natures power from the earth. Our bodies were designed for the clean stuff. Have something healthy that you enjoy drinking.

Now the best juicing combination for me is carrots and green apples, some times I add palmagranite. I know that the Gerson therapy says to use a juice presser, but I didn't feel like spending big bucks on a juice press. Instead I bought an Omega slow crushing juicer ($250). Maybe they have a better one now, but I think my machine is good quality, and I believe it works in a slightly similar fashion to the super expensive juice press.

I have a slice of apple, and then a piece of carrot. When they get crushed together they create a tasty combination. I just know that my body loves it. It's worth the extra money to buy a good quality crushing juicer, especially when you're juicing greens like kale and spinach.

When it comes to juicing greens, cheap spinning machines leave half the juice still trapped inside the pulp! Dig deep if you can, buy a quality juicer and get that good stuff out of the pulp.

Fill your system with good healthy liquid. Remember, you must complete the water equilibrium process before moving onto the next step.

Do not drink more than 4 glasses of water in 90 minutes, unless you are sweating and need extra hydration. If I reach the 4 glass mark and still haven't hit the bathroom for a pee, I stop drinking water; I know my kidneys are just being stubborn.

When you've reached water equilibrium, it's time to begin the cell dilation process.

Notes

(Note #5) ~ From page 25 – The Complete Book Of Juicing, Michael T. Murray, N.D. FORWORD By Jay Kordich, "The Juiceman". Prima Publishing copyright 1997 Page 236 ISBN: 0761511261

3 – Dilate

Turn on nature's cell washing machine!

This is my cell dilation theory. One day I believe science will discover that certain waste removal organs/cells do indeed dilate and flush from exposure to Cannabis. That detoxing with Cannabis does indeed dislodge and help to remove trapped toxic waste.

Maybe it's the relaxation caused by the tetrahydrocannabinol, which everyone knows as THC. THC is the stuff that gets people high. Maybe it's a natural reaction that happens when the body comes into contact with Cannabidiol, which everyone calls CBD. CBD does not get you high. THC and CBD's do different things, but both are found in varying levels of Cannabis medicine.

I believe all that happens when you use Cannabis is that certain cells in your body dilate/swell up ever so slightly, and then a short time later, the cell's diameter contracts back to regular size. I know dilation happens to the pupils in our eyes, and there's also a thirst that's triggered by something that's happening internally. I'm neither a scientist nor a doctor, but the same observations occur every time, with the same results, year after year.

Imagine a VERY slow 90-minute roller coaster ride where you only go up and down a very small hill while saying wooOOOooo. That's it, there's not much more to the story of what happens in real life when you use medical-grade Sativa Cannabis.

There's no doubt that Sativa strands of Cannabis work miracles for those of us who dilate and micro-cleanse the cells in our body. With a little medical grade Sativa Cannabis, I can gently encourage my cells to ever so slightly take in a tiny amount of freshly introduced moisture using its dilation properties.

Then after about 90 minutes when the cell's bloated diameter contracts, that gentle pressure slowly pushes out the cells waste. It creates a predictable wave/process that can be controlled and coordinated with other efforts to create the circumstances for my detox plan.

The dilation step also helps us to relax while the newly introduced liquid deep cleanses the body's passage ways and waste corridors. When people only use Cannabis to unwind, they miss a golden opportunity. Try "The Munchies Challenge," AKA Don's Super Flush light. Drink one glass of water fifteen minutes before dilating, and then another glass during the fifteen minutes after you've dilated.

You'll have clearer skin, cleaner kidneys, and better judgment, all from drinking two glasses of water at the correct time. If you relax with Cannabis, remember to try The Munchies Challenge the next time you dilate!

Anyone who has ever used Cannabis knows it causes dryness around the lips. Most people call it cotton mouth. While I'm aware that scientists have linked cotton mouth to certain receptors around the lips becoming activated by exposure to Cannabis; I believe your body also gets triggered into accommodating the dilation/swelling of more important cell areas throughout your system. Self

30

preservation kicks in, your body's default plan for survival from dehydration is set into motion.

Did you know that hunger is often mistaken for thirst? Hollywood sells the term "Munchies" and everyone starts eating when they use Cannabis. I say if you're properly hydrated you will not experience dry mouth with Cannabis. I say in the real world, munchies are just your body calling out for more water to help with the micro-cleansing dilation process.

I also believe the amount of toxin fighting you have going on in your body has a direct correlation to the level of happiness you experience. If your health is suffering, you'll be less happy. Hydrating with water makes things easier for your cells to remove toxic chemical compounds, your body has to fight less.

If dilation helps to cleanse and reduce the toxins in your brains cells, that would clear the path to less nerve stress on the brain. I see repair as the only cure for most stressed/blocked nerve connections, and dilation enhanced waste removal as the only catalyst for repair.

So I can either take a Cannabis supplement and drink water, or hope that one day they'll build microscopic robots that can clean up these blocked receptors. The choice is simple. Removing toxins from your brain fluids has to lead a person towards better health. It has to be the first step towards happier thinking.

When your system is breaking down, anything you can do to help your body work less gives more energy to the repair department. This is the whole story of medical

Cannabis for me. It calms my muscles and reduces the impact of stress. It's also there to help me get a good night's sleep without feeling groggy in the morning. It helps my body to detox and better remove waste. Because of these things, my system has more energy to fight disease.

Every garbage pail needs to be emptied and if nobody comes to pick up the garbage, it begins to back up. Backed up garbage slowly turns the waste corridor toxic, and then other corridors near by end up struggling as well. Slowly this ever-growing mass begins to show up on x-rays as darkness.

I believe that one day Cannabis will be looked upon with just a yawn, another one of those over the counter health supplements. It was only 200 years ago that people considered tomatoes to be poisonous. The world is starting to discover new things about the plants right in front of us.

There appears to be four levels of medical-grade Cannabis being produced for the public. There are different companies trying to get their brand names out into the minds of consumers, but vapor cartridge manufacturers provide very similar levels of THC and CBD in their combinations of the four types of medication.

I've thought about the best way to describe these four Cannabis medication levels and I think the strength of THC that gets a person high, is comparable to the level of intoxication a person experiences when consuming alcohol.

I will define the four levels of the Cannabis high, and suggest the equivalent level of alcohol needed to achieve an equal state of inebriation.

Every three second draw off of a vaporizer gives you about 2mg of vaporized Cannabis supplement. I believe two 3 second draws, five times a day is considered the moderate dosage at all four levels of THC strength.

One ingredient that people think does the most healing is called Cannabidiol, CBD's. Having been a musician for over 30 years, I've been around a lot of stuff, and today's medical grade Ruderalis and Sativa vaporizers work wonders for me.

Ruderalis is packed with CBD's and should be available to anyone at anytime. You don't get high from Ruderalis. It's the new vitamin C!!!

On the other side of the street are the people who just want to relax, and they're looking for THC. THC is the stuff that empties the mind and can put you off into a deep sleep without the drugged up hangover affect you get from taking sleeping pills.

As great as Indicas are, I think today's Indica strains are too strong for me; but God bless those who need them.

Funny thing how Sativa plants grow tall and have skinny leaves, and they keep me alert and thin; and the much shorter fat leafed Indica plants sedate me and causes me to gain weight.

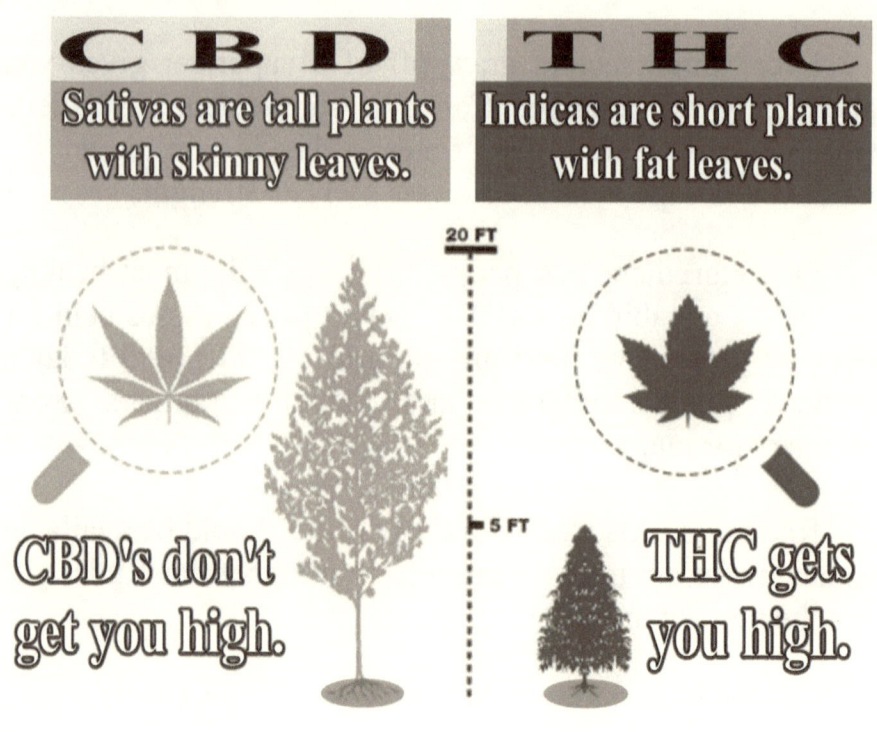

The four levels I see are:

Level 1 - Ruderalis - Insignificant THC – No feeling of getting high, equal to a spoon of beer. One strain called "Charlottes Web" is used by children to help control seizures. It's mostly used by those who only want the good CBD's from Cannabis, they're not interested in getting high.

There's no effect on a persons thinking or motor skills, and it's safe for anyone at any age. I believe Ruderalis should be sold in the vitamin section of every grocery store as a heath supplement.

Level 2 - Sativa - Small amounts of THC – A slight sense of relaxation, equal to 1-2 beers. No observable effects on thinking or motor skills, other than a smile. The euphoric producing properties in Sativa are weaker than Hybrids and Indicas, but it's packed with CBD's.

It's considered light stuff but it works miracles for me and many others who're associated with the health at home movement.

Level 3 - Hybrids - Moderate amount of THC – Nice deeper relaxation, equal to a bottle of wine. This is where growers try to create the perfect blend/mixture of CBD's and THC. Slight observable effects on thinking and motor skills. Lasts about 1-2 hours.

Level 4 - Indicas - Large amounts of THC – This is the stuff that will get you high! I am very sensitive to Indica strains. This stuff overwhelms my system and makes me a couch potato. Indicas do produce heavy observable effects on thinking and motor skills; but that only lasts for a couple of hours.

Think of these four levels of strength as four seating sections on a sailboat. The guy closest to the rudder is in control. Ruderalis is always sober and ready to steer the ship. Ruderalis doesn't get high.

Sativa is the next closest seat. Sativa people relax a little, but Sativa people are able to steer if needed. They don't get high.

Hybrids are that middle area between slight and heavy, where the moderate land for a blended mix of the Sativa's mild effect AND the stronger sedative effects from the Indica. The Hybrid passengers are more interested in just being a passenger, they're not there to steer.

Indica people are ready to drop anchor, they just want to relax and empty their thoughts for a couple of hours.

Here is an attempt at a graphic showing how I and most people I know would reasonably rate the four levels of intoxication from using Cannabis.

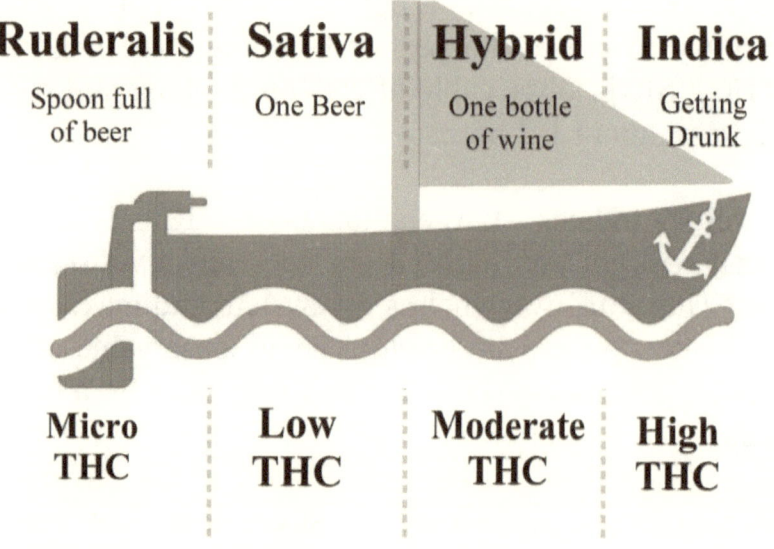

Ruderalis   **Sativa**   **Hybrid**   **Indica**

Spoon full of beer   One Beer   One bottle of wine   Getting Drunk

Micro THC   **Low THC**   **Moderate THC**   **High THC**

People who smoke huge bowls of very strong Indica at parties impress me as much as those who gulp big sips of whiskey straight from the bottle. There are no gateway drugs for YAHOO people; their excessive desires have more to do with escape than addiction. Using a large amount of Indica just overwhelms my body.

I think Indica strands of Cannabis are way to strong for first time users. But that's what the party crowd calls the "Good Stuff". I believe it's why some first timers have a bad experience with Cannabis, because they started out with stuff that was way too strong. I say instead of using THC filled Cannabis to get high, use CBD filled Cannabis to get healthy!

I am a legal medical marijuana user here in the state of Florida. I've dealt with stress and a medical issue ever since leaving the United States Navy in 1982. I joined straight out of high school like some other scouts I grew up with. During a basic training exercise mishap my left testicle was seriously injured. The doctors said it could take months for my body to repair the damage.

My commanding officer told me in rare cases like this, I would be honorably discharged, and sent home to heal instead of sitting around the hospital for 2-3 months. If my injury healed, I could rejoin as they would be happy to have me back.

It was peace time, it was the early 80's; and my term of service back then would have been a lot easier compared to what our military men and women have to deal with in Iraq and Afghanistan today. My commanding officer thanked me for my service and handed me my papers, shook my hand and wished me well.

Unfortunately for me, my injury never healed; I felt destroyed at the starting line. When you're a teenager and you loose your left nut, that trauma carries with you through life. Sativa Cannabis has helped me to live with the stress from my military medical issue. If you're a Veteran, and you struggle with anxiety, chronic pain or PTSD, I believe you'll find great relief with the low THC Ruderalis and Sativa strands of medical-grade Cannabis.

This is real life for those of us who supplement our health with medical-grade Cannabis. We're not actors trying to look cool in a movie. We're just average Americans working to improve our health as we get older.

In my opinion, with Sativas the mind has a tendency to seek out happier thoughts, to become more hopeful towards finding a positive answer. Sativa is for people who concentrate on problem solving, and Indicas are for people who want to forget about their problems.

I always smile when I hear the Eagles sing "Some dance to remember, some dance to forget." To me that says the whole story of Sativa and Indica. Sativa people like to think while Indica people like to empty their thoughts.

There are plenty of people out there who know the benefits of detoxing with Cannabis; and we're positive that there's absolutely nothing dangerous about Cannabis.

In fact, with all my experiences in life, and as a witness to the lives of others, I've never seen or thought of Cannabis as a gateway drug. I've always observed excessive alcohol as being the gateway to all hard drugs illegal and prescription.

I say most crack, meth, heroin, and other hard drug users start out as excessive drinkers. I also know a lot of normal acting people out there who use alcohol and prescription pills to blur their reality. For people in struggle, alcohol provides them with their first mental break.

When drinking, they're able to stop thinking about their unpleasant day-to-day reality. When sober, they feel powerless to cope with their positions in life, and the world they believe they're hopelessly locked into. They spend years poisoning their bodies with unhealthy living habits. There are no limits to how far people will go to dull their pain.

They become aware that the more they take, the more they can make themselves "feel" better. Then it's just mathematics. The increase in their pain brings on the need for an increase in blurring power. The greater the increase in desire for blurring out a painful reality, the more excessive a person becomes in his or her search for a higher high.

A lot of adults who drank excessively when they were young, remember most of their delinquent behavior being linked to alcohol. When I think back about my life as a young foolish teenager, I wish I'd been stoned instead of drunk.

I would have caused fewer struggles in my life, and would have been less of a pain in the ass to others. Struggle and stress in your brain create the first steps to using alcohol for comfort instead of celebration. Too much alcohol is the gateway drug.

But people still grin and shrug their shoulders when talking about excessive drinkers and chain smokers. It's an acceptable right to drink and smoke cigarettes in our society, yet both of these things cause degenerative diseases and cancer. They both kill you, but you can walk into any grocery store and buy as much as you want 365 days a year!

Those who stand vehemently against legalizing Cannabis, who drag their heels, who still demand that users be arrested, now only raise eyebrows. Their stance on harsh punishment only sparks more doubts about their other judgments.

But Times are changing. More people are quitting cigarettes and cutting out those after work drinks. They're switching over to Cannabis and chamomile, natures C & C, and they wake up feeling great. It's time to step back and take a deep breath; Cannabis is not poison, it's an incredible health supplement from a natural medicinal herb. It heals, and now Cannabis has been shown to help people with cancer.

The American Cancer Society acknowledges that some cancer is being cured with cannabinoids. I feel very comfortable saying, Cannabis and water helps the body to deep cleanse and flush out toxins, and that helps the repair department remove and replace cancerous cells.

"More recently, scientists reported that THC and other cannabinoids such as CBD slow growth and/or cause death in certain types of cancer cells growing in lab dishes. Some animal studies also suggest certain cannabinoids may slow growth and reduce spread of some forms of cancer." The American Cancer Society, Cancer.org (Note #6)

So if you become ill, there is hope. I believe the amount of time it takes for these degenerative diseases to materialize, is about the same amount of time it takes to kick them back to nothing or into a more controllable state.

It is possible to manage what happens in your body when detoxing with Cannabis. The next time you use Cannabis take the "Munchies Challenge". Drink a tall glass of water 15 minutes before and after, and then notice the pressure difference when you go to pee later.

Think about the pupil dilation properties of Cannabis, the unusual suddenness of cotton mouth, and the thirst that is so often mistaken for hunger. The results of my munchies challenge were that the munchies disappeared, no more cotton mouth, and a stronger pee stream!!!

I say to you now, if you only change your use of Sativa Cannabis to accommodate the hydration part for detoxing, in one year you'll be lighter and much healthier. Say goodbye to the munchies and say hello to clean water and fresh juice. Have fun AND get healthy.

OK OK, so now that you're hydrated and dilated, it's time to lay on the floor for the next 45 minutes and use that water to loosen up your body. Stretching can be fun exercise, and it helps to keep the body feeling younger and stronger.

When I say lets do some stretching I mean lets do some simple stretches, nothing that strains or pulls. If you feel discomfort, you're trying to hard. Go ahead and have one more glass of water during the stretch. I wait towards the end of my stretch routine before drinking water. Drink and pee says a me.

We all have different ways of stretching, and mine works the entire body from head to toe. If you have a pool with massage jets or a Jacuzzi, or jet tub, now is the best time to hit that and work your entire body.

Maybe get a massage from your significant other; it's mutually beneficial fun for couples to detox together. Team work makes "Detoxing With Cannabis" a breeze. But I do this alone and get on the floor and have a good stretch. Get a rug, a mat, or a big towel, but get off the couch and get on the floor!

One of the things I loved about Vietnam was how people young and old could easily get up and down from sitting on the floor. What might seem like a simple thing to do is actually very difficult for many people who're overweight. I like easy stretching, and slowly practicing getting up and down from the floor. Everything should be painless if you move slow and easy.

Do you want to unwind with my views on life? I have a 45-minute video of my stretch routine, and a 45-minute recording of relaxing music loaded with inspirational thoughts available at DonsSuperFlush.com.

While you're lying on the floor, also do some deep breathing exercises. Slowly take in a long breathe, and when you go to exhale, say the word "oooooofffff". Breathing out slowly while saying oooooffffff helps your body to relax; and I believe most animals understand the sound of oooofff.

So here is how you properly say oooooffffff. First say the word roof, and then say the word roof without the R.

Ooooooofffffff, it means the same thing to every human on earth, young and old! Everyone knows what you're feeling when you say it.

But back to business, you still have to get over that final hurdle. It's time to get ready for the full strength of Don's Super Flush. The big va voom, get ready to say OOOOOOOOOFFFFFFFFFFFF!

Notes

(Note #6) ~ From page 40 - The American Cancer Society

https://www.cancer.org/treatment/treatments-and-side-effects/complementary-and-alternative-medicine/marijuana-and-cancer.html

4 –Elimination

The coffee cleanse, it's not as bad as you think. After this, you'll wonder what all the fuss was about.

When will colon cleansing become part of our normal routine? A large number of people struggle with lower colon issues and for me nothing does the job like a good old coffee cleanse. The coffee cleanse dilates the bile duct to expand wide, and that means one big saturated flush.

I believe in this part of the Gerson therapy, because I think Dr. Max Gerson is correct in that the body first needs to be able to effectively remove its waste. If your waste removal organs are functioning properly, your body can work towards healing itself.

"For Max Gerson the right approach to practicing medicine involved regarding the human being as a whole unit that should be maintained in good health, if possible: how-ever, if sickness did occur, symptoms indicated some probable systemic weakness in the whole body. Thus Gerson's inclination as a healer was to search for ways to treat the total organism, not just address one or two of its many parts." Dr. Max Gerson, Healing The Hopeless, Howard Straus with Barbara Marinacci (Note #7)

The Gerson therapy by Dr. Max Gerson stood on the side of nutrition 100 years ago during the Pharmaceutical

VS Nutriceutical cancer curing debates. I personally like many of Dr. Max Gerson's observations and theories.

Dr. Max Gerson believed we could obtain better health by making things easier for our internal organs to remove their waste. It's time to wash that gathering place where everything comes out! The first time doing a coffee cleanse is the hardest, but after that it gets much much easier. Cleansing the lower colon is nothing new. It's been practiced for thousands of years by many famous healers.

In the Dead Sea scrolls Jesus refers to a lower colon cleanse as "The Angel of water". These people who took the time to cleanse themselves on the inside, lead happier and healthier lives on the outside. When Jesus cleansed people of their sins, did the translators mean to say toxins?

Learn to cleanse yourself; here is how my plan unfolds for Friday night. The Friday night cleansing gets everything loosened up for Saturday morning. First you hydrate to fill up your body's water tank. Then dilate to wash the cells with fresh moisture. Then eliminate with a coffee flush, and that clears the path for your body's night work.

About an hour to an hour and a half after I finish the evening portion, I usually have a very strong pee. After that strong pee, that's when I quick hydrate and dilate for the night work. I let the kidneys kick out any of that last waste they had laying around before dilating. At the end of this chapter I give you a list of everything you'll need for doing the coffee cleanse from start to finish. There's no need to take notes, it's already in here. ☺

In the morning when you wake up it's always a good habit to gargle with water and brush your teeth before drinking or eating anything for breakfast. Your mouth makes some pretty funky stuff while you sleep. Why would you want that muck going into your system? Only let healthy stuff into your stomach.

While you're sleeping your body will work to fill up the elimination path with more waste. So I wake up on Saturday morning, and do a quick tooth brushing and rinse. Then I Hydrate for half an hour with one glass of juice and one water. Then I do a coffee cleanse Elimination, and after I'm all cleaned up, I drink a glass of water to hydrate and dilate. So lets define the three parts of Don's Super Flush, and the order they should be done in.

Hydrate – Achieve water equilibrium in your body. Either drink all water, or one juice early and then the rest should be water. The reason I say juice first is because you want to make absolutely sure your body is getting that fresh nutrition, that's why juice is #1.

Dilate – Stretch and shrink the diameter of your important cells with your favorite strand of Sativa Cannabis. I like and suggest Sativa. When you infuse fresh moisture into the cells, it gently pushes out toxins later on the contraction side of that ride.

Eliminate – Flush out the lower intestine with a 20 minute coffee cleanse. Without coffee it's just an enema. It's the oil that comes out from boiling the coffee grinds that make the miracle happen.

Friday Night I usually start around 7:00PM

Hydrate – Most times I'm already well hydrated from the day. I know it's Friday, and I'm going to cleanse, so I drink tea all day.

Dilate – I dilate and then stretch for 45 minutes, keep drinking water.

Eliminate – 20 minutes for the cleanse, and 15 minutes for the flush.

Hydrate – I drink a glass of chamomile tea every two hours until I go to sleep. I may have to get up and pee during the night, but that's just part of the price you pay when you want to do your best!

Dilate – An hour after the elimination, I usually have a strong pee, and that's when I dilate for the night work. If you haven't had the urge to pee, don't worry, go ahead and dilate after your first glass of water or chamomile tea. Make sure to have your coffee ready for the morning.

Saturday Morning I start around 10AM

Brush your teeth and gargle with water before you begin.

Quick Hydrate – One glass of juice and one water over 40 minutes.

Eliminate – 20 minutes for the cleanse, and 15 minutes for the flush.

Quick Hydrate – One glass of juice or water over 30 minutes.

Dilate – An hour after the elimination, I usually have a strong pee, and that's when I dilate for the final cell wash.

The difference in the sequence for Saturday morning is because your body just worked all night refilling the elimination path back up with toxic sludge. We want to move out as much toxic waste as possible before calling upon the cells to dilate.

So Saturday morning a quick hydrate to make sure the coffee cleanse is not absorbed. Then do the coffee cleanse and flush. An hour after you're all cleaned up, it's just one last dilation. That last dilation cell wash will be flushed out later with your normal elimination cycle. Also stretching is not mandatory on Saturday mornings, but it's a great way to get loosened up for the weekend!

It takes time to set up and prepare for a coffee cleanse, so here's how I do it. First let's make a pot of coffee earlier in the day so it's ready for later. Go ahead and fill up your enema bag with water, and when it's full, pour that into the pitcher.

Mark that water line on the pitcher with a permanent marker. Now you know how much coffee you'll need in order to fill the enema bag. Then you can pour the pitcher into your coffee pot and you'll know that level as well. Leave a small reference mark scratch with a screwdriver or fork by the handle area.

OK, so most people want to know how much and what kind. I use regular ground coffee, and I like to add 3 heaping table spoons into every quart of water.

I only put half as much water as I need when starting to make the coffee. Later when it cools I will add more water to the pot so it's filled to the correct level. I set the stove to slightly above medium and turn the timer on for 20 minutes.

REMEMBER, when coffee begins to boil in a pot, it foams up FAST. And if your coffee boils over it's going to make a big mess, don't rush the process. Play it safe, set the stove to just a hair above medium, it shouldn't boil over at that setting. After 10 minutes the coffee begins to boil, and then after 20 minutes it's done.

I boil my coffee in the afternoon, and then keep a lid on the pot until I'm ready. You can boil two separate pots of coffee at the same time; one for the night and the other for the morning. But I like to make the second pot after I finish the night cleanse. Your coffee will not spoil, it's OK for coffee to sit on the stove overnight.

So when I'm ready to start the coffee cleanse, I like to check the temperature to make sure it's just right. Some people say it should be just below 105 degrees. I think it should be warm to the touch of the BACK of my hand. There is a difference in the level of sensation to both sides of my hand when it comes to feeling temperature; and the back of my hand seems more accurate for finding my comfort level.

If the coffee is to hot to touch with the back of your hand, you must wait for it to cool down. Never cleanse with hot coffee. So now that you've got the temperature right, slightly warm but not too hot, it's best to get the coffee from the pot into something more manageable. I take the coffee and pour it through a fine strainer into the pitcher.

When I have the right amount, I put a plastic funnel into the enema bag opening, and pour the coffee through the funnel. As the pitcher gets closer to being empty, you'll notice the stream becoming more and more filled with super fine particles of coffee grinds. Leave that stuff in the pitcher. Small particles of coffee grinds can clump together to cause problems for the enema tip.

So before I put the bag onto my transport tray, I hold the tip end low inside the empty pitcher and the bag higher, and quickly open and close the locking clasp to force out any air in the hose.

If you don't do this you will push air into your lower colon. I don't think air is bad, I just think coffee is better. So when coffee comes out of the tip I click the nozzle lock shut, and then place it onto my transport tray. The only time the hose clasp should be unlocked, is when you want it to be unlocked. Keep it locked at all other times.

It's very important to get an enema kit with a good locking clamp. I have put together everything you need in one package, and it's available on DonsSuperFlush.com. Or you can just print the free PDF list from the web site and get what you need, which ever makes you happy. So once the enema's on the transport tray, I do a quick clean up in the kitchen before heading to my bathroom, or lying area.

Tile, Marble and Terrazzo flooring make great surfaces to lay down on, but stay away from doing this on carpet or wood parquet. One day you're going to have a small mishap, the enema bag hose pops off, you just can't hold the coffee in, something will go wrong with the locking clasp, things happen.

So prepare now and reduce the impact of a potential event. I lay down on one towel, and have a 2nd one near by. I have my area set up with my tray, my clock to time myself, and my back up towel ready at hand, everything is within reach.

So there you are lying on your towel, you've already put lubrication on the tip and its destination. So you insert the tip, and then pop the hose locking clasp open. Then grab the bag and hold it high. You can accomplish insertion, unlocking, and bag holding with the same hand.

As the coffee cleanse flows in, you'll begin to feel very relaxed. A calm sensation slowly takes over your body. Be careful, the short enema tip can fall out if there's pressure. Have your towel ready, and don't panic, it's only coffee.

Many of you will feel a slight emotional release during the first cleanse. It's hard to explain the feeling of toxicity leaving your body. Your organs may have given up a long time ago. This sudden relief makes your system wonder what's going on.

I felt it my first time, like a sudden untying of knots in my stomach. You feel like shouting Hallelujah because your system is immediately amazed that bad stuff actually got removed. You wouldn't be surprised to hear some tiny toy you swallowed as a kid plop out when you go to flush the cleanse.

The bottom line is that you first timers shouldn't be nervous if you find yourself getting all emotional. Some people cry, some people sneeze or get a runny nose, but most people recognize the moment when a big clump of toxins is leaving their body.

Now when most people hear the words coffee retention enema they start thinking no way. But at 50 years old, I either deal with my health now, or wait until I'm in my 60's and medication becomes part of my diet.

So in your body you have 100's of different veins, muscles and bones. Now imagine that each of them has a garbage pail located on the corner where the vein meets the next bigger vein. Every cell of every organ has a system of taking in the good stuff and getting rid of its waste.

If time goes by and a garbage pail doesn't get emptied, that garbage pail AREA gets backed up. The worker cells keep bringing waste as close as they can to the garbage area, but nothing comes to take it away. Nothing is moving out of that area of the organ. That street gets backed up, then a couple of blocks near by start backing up, and then the whole neighborhood becomes filled with trash.

I believe similar toxins that float around the body, end up congregating around specific organs. Unique toxins are naturally drawn to organs that struggle with their removal. The organ is unable to do anything on it's own. Nature has never encountered these man-made toxins before.

The body has no internal dilation flushing process to assist with the removal of these laboratory created chemical compounds. I believe these toxins just float in like all the other similar toxins did before, and that organ begins to strain from the growing pile.

A garbage pail that is never emptied begins to rot. Remember me talking about those x-rays showing organs backing up and becoming diseased? I think if those organs could better remove their waste, to micro-flush, they would once again function properly. Together with Hydration and Dilation, the coffee flush helps to keep me and my engine running smoothly down the center of the road.

Unfortunately some people wait too long before trying to turn the steering wheel. Their health struggles to maneuver back into the correct direction. But when that third tire goes over the edge of the cliff, don't bother hitting the breaks.

That 4th tire isn't gonna do anything but screech and squeal. Some times the very last breath of that 4th tire smells like alcohol and cigarettes; but no matter the cause, all 4th tires going over the cliff yell the same thing, "Why Me."

This is usually the moment when YAHOO people suddenly want to get off the highway, but it's too late because they've already traveled beyond the point of no return. They look back through their review mirror staring at the last exit they passed, and they're not smiling.

But what if they turned the wheel just a little sooner. What if that highway sign read:

Would you have stopped to look your car over, maybe taken some time to fix a few things up?

I believe the inability of the body to effectively remove its waste is the most preventable cause of degenerative diseases and cancer. Pesticides, herbicides, hormone additives, neutralizers, stabilizers, if you're like most people, you've had your fair share of unhealthy processed foods and sugar drinks.

And that sludge piles up; layer on top of layer until it clogs your garbage pail shut. When one garbage pail is covered, the sludge moves onto the next one; and why not, you're not doing anything to stop it.

I've had much thought and discussion with others on the subject of fear. So which is worse, the disease, or the fear of having the disease. Which causes more harm to the body?

I say the FEAR alone of having a disease makes you sicker. Norman Cousins wondered about thought itself and asked the question:

"Is it possible that love, hope, faith, laughter, confidence, and the will to live have therapeutic value? Do chemical changes occur only on the downside?" Anatomy Of An Illness As Perceived By The Patient, by Norman Cousins (Note #8)

"The doctor knows that it is the prescription slip itself, even more than what is written on it, that is often the vital ingredient for enabling a patient to get rid of whatever is ailing him." Anatomy Of An Illness As Perceived By The Patient, by Norman Cousins. (Note #9)

Max Gerson also believed it the power of positive thought.

"If patients believed that a cure could be effected, they would cooperate with the treatment and not spend their time worrying. Gerson had already learned that the stress caused by fretting about the slow progress or lack of improvement itself generated toxic chemicals in the body that could stop the healing process." Dr. Max Gerson, Healing The Hopeless Howard Straus with Barbara Marinacci. (Note #10)

But you didn't get sick over night. What makes you think it's going to end tomorrow, what's the rush? I bet 90% of everything that kills us, does it faster if we continue living the way that brought it on.

How about taking a deep breath (and a little self-responsibility) and slowly begin to change the direction of your physical condition by gradually cutting down on the habits that are contributing to your health issues.

What about the commercials touting the benefits of a new drug on the market. Then a couple of years later those same drugs are in commercials again, but this time they're being touted by class-action lawyers looking for complainants.

In Anatomy Of An Illness As Perceived By The Patient by Norman Cousins, he states *"The history of medicine is replete with accounts of drugs and modes of treatment that were in use for many years before it was recognized that they did more harm than good."* (Note #11)

I think a lot of people have destroyed their lives with medication. Sometimes when I see the long list of side affects mentioned on TV commercials, it sounds to me like you'd be better off just living with the disease. But for most of us it's not the medicines we take that are killing us, it's the processed foods we eat every day.

Most people have horrible diets. I had 30 years of bad eating, canned and boxed dead empty food. But amazing things start to happen when you take care of cleaning out those old garbage pails. I believe if you assist your body with this regiment, your health will improve as toxic waste loses its dominance in the soluble composition of your body's chemistry.

From reading this book you will be able to imagine the process, and from that you will gain the confidence to actually make the coffee cleanse happen. The more toxins you're able to get out, the higher your level of good health becomes. That's why you're reading this book. You know you can do better, and a 20 minute coffee cleanse does miracles for the body.

So you're laying down on the floor on your right side, and you've just finished letting in all the coffee. You snap the lock closed and put the empty bag onto the transport tray. Later on you'll bring it with you into the bathroom to put inside the shower. The shower is a great place to wash everything, and you'll be using it again in the morning.

For the first couple of times I did the whole 20 minutes laying on my right side. Then as I became more comfortable with cleansing I was able to switch sides more easily. So now I lay on my right side for 10 minutes, and then on my left side for 10 minutes. Get used to cleansing before you start rolling around on the floor.

But I NEVER, never get up from the floor if I feel pressure. Now some day I know the dam might spring a small leak, and that's what the spare towel is for; but no pressure means no problems. You'll be OK if you have an accident. Relax, it's a simple clean up.

There will be times when you feel slight cramps in your stomach, some people say it feels like gas. This is normal and I just wiggle around a little bit with a five second countdown. 5,4,3,2,1, and that seems to help me move through the discomfort. If I lay still and try to wait the pressure out, it always seems to grow. A wiggle will get you through those pressure build ups.

But most times after 20 minutes I just carefully get up, move the tray into the shower, and have a seat on the toilet. Make sure you prepare your toilet for when you're going to release the coffee cleanse. I put the seat up and place toilet paper around the back. Sit right on the rim, not the seat, there's hardly any clean up afterwards.

Try not to use too much toilet paper. You don't want to clog up your pipes with a big ball of cotton. It takes me about 15-20 minutes to get the flush out. Have patience; get out as much as you can. The release usually happens in 2 – 4 waves. Don't Rush The Flush!

VERY IMPORTANT :(After you've finished showering, cleaning and putting your cloths on, if you feel like you're going to fart, it's not a fart. Go back and have a seat on the toilet. It's a good idea to rinse yourself after each time going back; the very last stuff coming out came from the deepest places.

When I was a kid and you broke one lose, the big fart joke was to ask everyone around, "Hey do farts have lumps?" That was funny when I was a kid, but as an adult finishing up a detox regiment, well it's still funny but you have to take one simple precaution. Just use a little toilet paper to create a barrier between you and your clothes for an hour or two.

Some times while you're releasing the cleanse it feels like the coffee has gotten warmer than when you started. What you're feeling is the toxins leaving your body. Some say it's old heavy metals coming into contact with your outer skin. This is normal and nothing to worry about; actually if it happens, it should be celebrated!

My neighbor once asked me, can someone become addicted to coffee cleansing. Maybe, but I believe the desire/necessity of coffee cleansing lowers as the concentration levels of toxins in your body decreases. The more you get out from successful detoxing, the less you'll have to do in the future.

How often you cleanse is all dependant on how much you need to fix and repair. I say it's like being addicted to brushing your teeth. Imagine what your smile would look like if you only cleaned your mouth with napkins for 30 years.

Sometimes you get rid of so much backed up waste that you don't have a movement for a day or two. I've been through this before, and it's not so bad when it happens. My solution to irregular movements is simple, I eat popcorn every night of the week.

When you detox with Cannabis, you want to stay regular AND also keep those toxins moving out of the body. Plain tasteless popcorn is what I eat, and it never lets me down in the morning. Popcorn turns into a gentle scrubbing sponge that pushes everything through your intestinal tract. I say if you want to live long, ya gotta eat some popcorn!

So I want to go over the list of everything you'll need for the cleanse, and explain what each item is for. It's good to be familiar with all the components before you start.

1 – Cooking pot to boil coffee - Fill the enema bag with water, then pour into the pitcher and use a magic marker to draw your full pitcher line. Then pour that into the pot and

use a screwdriver or fork to make a little scratch showing the level of water needed in the pot.

2 - Spring water or good filtered water - I filter my own water for everything, one of those filter pitchers works great for me. But a gallon of spring water from the store makes some people feel better.

3 - Coffee – Regular coffee with caffeine is the winner. Do not get decaffeinated. I use three tablespoons per quart of water. You don't need organic or expensive coffee. What ever the store has that is regular ground coffee, that's what you're looking for. Remember to only fill the pot up half way when making coffee, because later on you'll add more water into the pot to meet the line.

4 – Fine Strainer – This is for catching the grinds while transferring the coffee from the pot to the pitcher. You must strain the coffee grinds to keep them from clogging up the tip of the enema hose.

5 - Pitcher/Container - The pitcher makes it easier for you to pour the coffee into the enema bag. Remember to use a permanent marker to show the line for a full enema bag.

When you're almost finished pouring out the coffee, you'll see the finer grains starting to show as it gets close to empty. Leave that stuff in the pitcher.

6 - Funnel – To help pour coffee from the pitcher into the enema bag. It's just easier to use a funnel.

7 - Enema Kit – I say when you're experienced, use 1 quart for a small person, 2 for an average person, and 3 quarts for a giant person. Until you get some experience you should start with half the amounts of liquid for your coffee cleanse.

Let your body get used to cleansing before filling your stomach up with liquid. Then after you've done it a few times, you can increase the amount of coffee for the cleanse. Remember to keep the hose clamp locked until you decide to open it.

8 - Tray for holding everything – I use one of those huge plastic serving trays from the dollar store. It's easier to transport everything to my lying area, and then into the shower.

9 – Clock or Timer – You need to know how long you've been holding that coffee cleanse.

10 - Two big towels - One to lay down on the floor with, and the other near by as a back up for sudden mishaps.

11 - Toilet area – I lift the seat up and toilet paper the back area. Take the time to prepare the back of your toilet and everything will be OK. Sit right on the rim, it makes cleaning a breeze. Don't clog your pipes with toilet paper!!!

That's everything I use to do a coffee cleanse. When you have all of these items, you'll sail straight through the coffee cleansing part of this therapy.

So from start to finish that's how Don's Super Flush works. In the next chapter I talk about a few other things like diet and exercise, but it's Don's Super Flush that makes the magic happen. The coffee cleanse is the last hurdle before the finish line.

When you know what to do, and you've got everything set up, it gets pretty simple. All you need is a little time for yourself. And as I said in the beginning, "It takes courage to step past this line for the first time. After that, you'll wonder what all the fuss was about."

Ten years ago I chose to start fixing myself back up, because when I looked around at other people, I was able to see who did and didn't make it back to good health.

There are two extreme health paths and not much in the middle. One is huge and filled with people that have horrible health and suffer every day, and the other is a thinner path filled with people who have good health and happiness.

Don's Super Flush, create your own first class ticket to a lifetime of good health!

Notes

(Note #7) ~ From page 45 -Dr. Max Gerson, Healing The Hopeless, Howard Straus with Barbara Marinacci, Kensington Books copyright 2001   Page 77   ISBN: 0976018616

(Note #8) ~ From page 56 – Anatomy Of An Illness As Perceived By The Patient, by Norman Cousins. W.W. Norton & Company, Inc. Page 37 ISBN: 0393041905

(Note #9) ~ From page 56 – Anatomy Of An Illness As Perceived By The Patient, by Norman Cousins. W.W. Norton & Company, Inc. Page 37 ISBN: 0393041905

(Note #10) ~ From page 56 - Dr. Max Gerson, Healing The Hopeless, Howard Straus with Barbara Marinacci, Kensington Books copyright 2001   Page 84   ISBN: 0976018616

(Note #11) ~ From page 57 – Anatomy Of An Illness As Perceived By The Patient, by Norman Cousins. W.W. Norton & Company, Inc. Page 40 ISBN: 0393041905

5 – Exercise, Diet And Quit Smoking

"Every human being is the author of his own health or disease." - Buddha

Everyone has an exercise program that they like, and detoxing with Cannabis will help your routine to work the way you wished it would. The problem with exercise is if you're not detoxing, then you're just moving those water soluble toxins around your body.

Your mind begins to relax when you put on a couple of pounds, the body LOVES making fat! Your body grabs these toxins that are floating around and sticks them into the new fat. As the toxins lessen in the fluids moving through your body, the stress alarms shut off, and with each bit of chocolate the body says oooooffffff. But when you get back into exercising and burn away that new fat, you hit that toxic layer again; and those concentrated toxin loaded fat cells kick back hard and fast.

You suddenly find yourself angry and frustrated, but every aspect of your life is fine. You ask yourself why do I feel this way, and the answer is simple, it's old toxins. You just hit that dirty layer carrying all the extra toxins from your last failed diet and exercise program. There's only so long your body is willing to fight a losing battle.

I believe this swirling mass of water soluble toxins wears your body's enthusiasm down. Endless struggle forces the body to give up the desire to fight. It surrenders but with a great protest that lingers in your background thinking.

This is the struggle with exercise, and once you start incorporating Don's Super Flush into your health routine, you'll get rid of those old toxins once and for all!!!

For me, my favorite exercise is to slowly bicycle everywhere, and I leisurely walk/jog at the park and on the beach. Now that I have my health back I can get outside five days a week, and I stay fairly active working around the house and yard.

I think the best exercise to start with is stretching. I turned my garage into a home gym. I bought a big area rug, got some light hand weights, and built a pull up bar. I go in there when ever I have time, and I spend most of it on the floor stretching to the radio.

I did P90X a couple of times, but I was never able to keep up with their full workout, and at best I was only able to do half of Ab Ripper X. It's good to sit there and get your body used to the P90X exercises, no one is watching; just do the best you can without hurting or straining yourself. I enjoyed just following along with the video, slowly learning to do each exercise correctly.

In time you can learn to do a lot of perfect push ups, and perfect sit ups. I bought some stretch bands and wrapped them around my pull up bar to practice doing pull ups, and after three years I was able to do a chin up again.

Start getting your body into the habit of doing exercise. I was never in a rush for results, I knew it was going to be a long time before I looked good in a t-shirt. Slow and steady was the way I put the weight on, and that's the way I took it off. My goal was a worthy ideal; I wanted to see what nature intended for me to look like before I got too old to try.

Most people want to lose the weight overnight. But what you really need is a long-term plan for slow change. You slowly changed to become what you are now, how about a better version of you in the near future.

Because whether you take the time to change slowly or not, the future is coming. One day you'll be three years older, and the choice you make right here right now will decide whether you become lighter, healthier and happier.

Here is a simple three-year plan for losing weight. Your time frame might move quicker or slower, but it's important to just start moving yourself towards a healthier lifestyle now. First stop drinking sugar drinks during the day for a month, then the second month cut them out completely. Drink water, sparkling water with lemon and teas.

Try to get down on the floor for three 45-minute stretch sessions a week. Whether its the floor area in front of your TV or an empty room, it doesn't matter, just get on the floor and stretch. Don't work up a sweat, move slow, relax while you stretch.

As to the question of how often should you do the Don's Super Flush. I think for me, once a week with light exercise is enough. But there are times when I exercise a lot and do it twice a week. That's night and morning. And when I'm juice fasting for the entire work week, I do it once a day in the morning. People on the Gerson therapy who are fighting cancer and other degenerative diseases do the coffee cleanse 3-5 times a day, seven days a week, until their health returns!

"Enemas of boiled coffee are taken by the patient as needed, as frequently as every four hours throughout the day, for their ability to alleviate pain, detoxify, and improve nutritional condition (see chapter 12). Occasional nighttime enemas are suggested in special cases. The Gerson Therapy, Charlotte Gerson and Morton Walker, (Note #12)

Don't try to start doing everything tomorrow, turn your steering wheel slowly over two months. Maybe do Don's Super Flush twice a week, twice a month or even twice a year. We are all different, and you will find your level when you start.

This is not a race, some people may want to speed their changes up, while others may want to slow things down. Don't rush yourself into taking on more than you can handle. Start slowly, phase out sugar drinks from your diet, and stretch three times a week.

After six months of that, change your morning diet to be all fruit or anything else from the earth you might enjoy for breakfast. The goal is to have your first meal of the day come from nature and not a factory. Eating healthy for two out of three meals a day ended up being the winning combination for me.

Also learn to chew your food longer. The more you chew the easier it is for your body to absorb the nutrients. Barely chewed big clumps of food can temporarily clog up the intestines. Next time you put food into your mouth, count the amount of times you chew before swallowing. Make a conscious effort to chew longer, TRY!!!

So after six months you've stopped drinking soda, you are exercising three times a week, and you are starting your day with a healthy meal. Then for the next three months clean up your lunch, and then around the 9th month start walking or bicycling.

That's year one, continue along this new direction for the next two additional years and you'll lose 30 pounds a year. No problem.

We have start calendars on the web site for what ever month you start. Just go to DonsSuperFlush.com and download the PDF for the month you started; and you'll have all the information you need to make it through the year. You can hang it on your fridge or just put it somewhere by your desk to see everyday as a reminder.

Instead of checking off days, you check off months. We're going to move slow and steady over the next three years, heading straight towards our goal. The focus is more on the finish line rather than how fast we can get there. Because when you pass the finish line, you want to smoothly continue moving towards the land of good health and happiness; that should be your life long goal!!!

The Japanese use the word Kaizen, and it's about making yourself a little better each day. Small changes add up over time, this I could do, and I'm telling you it works. Deliberate changes, little changes, just be aware of what you're eating and drinking. Look to eat and drink things that come from the earth.

I don't have much will power, everyone thinks I do, but I don't. I discovered that if I stretched out my weight loss plan, I could do this all over three years, and that's what I did. It's not hard to lose a hundred pounds when you're doing it over three years. This I know for a fact!

I drink beer and wine on the weekends, and live a fairly quiet life. I tried veganism, didn't like it. Then I went pescetarianism, but I wanted more than seafood. Simple moderation seemed to provide me with the most fulfilling diet.

Monday through Friday I have fruit and maybe a coconut for breakfast, a salad for lunch, and a reasonably healthy dinner. But on Saturday and Sunday, I enjoy what ever I like, even dessert!

I just don't go overboard anymore, I've become more aware of what I put into my system. I do occasionally eat junk food about once a month. I love chocolate, but I learned to slowly control my sugar addictions. I also stopped drinking coffee. It might wake me up in the morning, but it doesn't make me feel healthy like green tea does.

I tried everything, read book after book, and experimented with dozens of different vitamins and supplements before Don's Super Flush magically came together. A good multi vitamin, B12 , iron, and plenty of vitamin C, this works for me. Do some research on vitamin C, I think it's the most valuable vitamin!

Some times when you mix vitamins and supplements their combinations can make your stomach feel a little upset. Whenever you want to test a new vitamin or supplement, try it after lunch by itself to see if it has any adverse affects. Then if it's OK put it in with your morning line up.

That's what I did for my diet and exercise, and now I'll share with you how I quit smoking cigarettes. The more I detoxed the easier it was for me to quit smoking cigarettes.

I used the Nicoderm cq 21 mg patches to help break the addiction; you're not kicking the habit, you're breaking an addiction. I tried the nicotine gum but that just didn't work for me. Some people love the gum, but it was the patches that helped me to slowly quit cigarettes.

In the morning I would put on a patch, and then after finishing my day I would take the patch off. So Monday-Friday during the day I used the patch, and then for evenings and weekends I smoked. It's interesting how much less I smoked when I made a conscious effort to recognize each time I lit one up.

Within two weeks of slowly increasing the length of time for wearing the patch, and with continued deep cleansing, I was able to completely stop smoking cigarettes just by wearing the patch.

I took evening primrose oil and drank chamomile tea every morning when I started; and then drank chamomile tea a couple more times throughout the day. Primrose oil and chamomile tea helps to take the edge off of quitting smoking, I'd say by half, but you gotta keep flushing out those toxins.

I was doing Don's Super Flush twice a week. Tuesday night and Wednesday morning, and then again Friday night and Saturday morning. It wasn't that bad, I actually felt happier with each cleanse, and I'm not kidding! Some days when you are just starting to quit, you feel like you could chew through shoe leather.

Then after two weeks I cut down the dosage to half a patch, and then two weeks later to a quarter. Then one day I forgot to put the patch on, and the primrose oil and chamomile tea got me through the day.

After a couple of months there were times when I wanted to smoke, and I would put on an 1/8th of a patch. That tiny little bit actually helped. I also wore a quarter patch if I went to a party or bar where people would be smoking. Don't smoke and wear the patch at the same time, that's just asking for a heart attack.

After three months the cravings were pretty much gone, even after a couple of drinks in a smoke filled bar. I just wasn't a smoker anymore. I didn't just quit, I also kept up with my weekly detox cleansing, and that gave my body the strength to stop once and for all. You gotta do the flush to get those toxins out, and cigarettes are loaded with toxins!

I try to do a yearly juice fast for five days, and that's something you need to work up to. If you're interested in doing a long juice fast, try to get through one day first. It's not as easy as you think. With a little online research you can find a juice recipe that works for you.

Once again let's review Don's Super Flush.

The Friday night cleansing gets everything loosened up for Saturday morning. First you hydrate to fill up your body's water tank. Then dilate to wash the cells with fresh moisture. Then eliminate with a coffee flush, and that clears the path for your body's night work.

About an hour to an hour and a half after I finish the evening portion of Don's Super Flush, I usually have a very strong pee. After that strong pee, that's when I quick hydrate and dilate for the night work. I let the kidneys kick out any of that last waste they had laying around before dilating. At the end of this chapter I give you a list of everything you'll need for doing the coffee cleanse from start to finish. There's no need to take notes, it's already in here. ☺

In the morning when you wake up it's always a good habit to gargle with water and brush your teeth before drinking or eating anything for breakfast. Your mouth makes some pretty funky stuff while you sleep. Why would you want that muck going into your system? Only let healthy stuff into your stomach.

While you're sleeping your body will work to fill up the elimination path with more waste. So I wake up on Saturday morning, and do a quick tooth brushing and rinse. Then I Hydrate for half an hour with one glass of juice and one water. Then I do a coffee cleanse Elimination, and after I'm all cleaned up, I drink a glass of water to hydrate and dilate. So lets define the three parts of Don's Super Flush, and the order they should be done in.

Hydrate – Achieve water equilibrium in your body. Either drink all water, or one juice early and then the rest should be water. The reason I say juice first is because you want to make absolutely sure your body is getting that fresh nutrition, that's why juice is #1.

Dilate – Stretch and shrink the diameter of your important cells with your favorite strand of Sativa Cannabis. When you infuse fresh moisture into the cells, it gently pushes out toxins later on the contraction side of that ride.

Eliminate – Flush out the lower intestine with a 20 minute coffee cleanse. Without coffee it's just an enema. It's the oil that comes out from boiling the coffee grinds that make the miracle happen.

Friday Night I usually start around 7:00PM

Hydrate – Most times I'm already well hydrated from the day. I know it's Friday, and I'm going to cleanse, so I drink tea all day.

Dilate – I dilate and then stretch for 45 minutes, keep drinking water.

Eliminate – 20 minutes for the cleanse, and 15 minutes for the flush.

Hydrate – I drink a glass of chamomile tea every two hours until I go to sleep. I may have to get up and pee during the night, but that's just part of the price you pay when you want to do your best!

Dilate – An hour after the elimination, I usually have a strong pee, and that's when I dilate for the night work. If you haven't had the urge to pee, don't worry, go ahead and dilate after your first glass of water or chamomile tea. Make sure to have your coffee ready for the morning.

Saturday Morning I start around 10AM

Brush your teeth and gargle with water before you begin.

Quick Hydrate – One glass of juice and one water over 40 minutes.

Eliminate – 20 minutes for the cleanse, and 15 minutes for the flush.

Quick Hydrate – One glass of juice or water over 30 minutes.

Dilate – An hour after the elimination, I usually have a strong pee, and that's when I dilate for the final cell wash.

The difference in the sequence for Saturday morning is because your body just worked all night refilling the elimination path back up with toxic sludge. We want to move out as much toxic waste as possible before calling upon the cells to dilate.

So Saturday morning a quick hydrate to make sure the coffee cleanse is not absorbed. Then do the coffee cleanse and flush. An hour after you're all cleaned up, it's just one last dilation.

That last dilation cell wash will be flushed out later with your normal elimination cycle. Also stretching is not mandatory on Saturday mornings, but it's a great way to get loosened up for the weekend!

That's it, this regiment plus eating healthy and basic exercising is what did it for me; and now you know how I lost 100 pounds, quit smoking, and got my health back. I hope you're able to experience the same level of success that I've had in turning my health around. Remember that life is long, and the best thing you could ever invest in, will always be yourself!!!

If you benefit from my work, please purchase a printed copy from DonsSuperFlush.com to balance out our exchange and keep good Karma flowing.

It also makes for an interesting coffee table conversation piece. When you want to watch your guests raise an eyebrow ☺

Also Don's Super Flush T-Shirt will make you an instant hit at ANY party! You know you want one or two, maybe three!!!

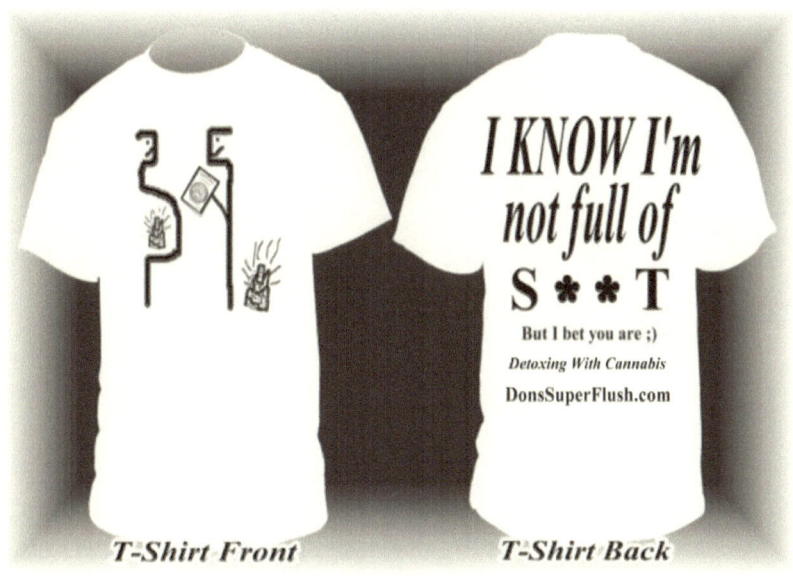

T-Shirt Front   **T-Shirt Back**

OK, if you didn't get the cartoon, one of them has read my book. I know no one is going to buy that t-shirt. But I just started laughing my ass off when I drew it; and then I thought, why not, maybe it's so stupid somebody else might get a kick out of it.

But I have a favor to ask, as small as the chances are of the following ever happening in this world; IF, if you ever see anyone wearing that t-shirt, I hope you smile and give them two thumbs up while saying, "Don's Super Flush!"

T-shirt aside, please do mention "Don's Super Flush" to your friends and family on your social media accounts.

That's it, bye bye for now. Until next time, have fun, be safe, and remember that you are the goose that lays your own golden eggs. Take care of the goose!!!

Don Endriss out!

Notes

(Note #12) ~ From page 68 – The Gerson Therapy, Charlotte Gerson and Morton Walker, Kensington Books copyright 2001   Page 95   ISBN: 1-57566-628-6

Some books worth considering.

Law of Success: The Original Unedited Edition– Napoleon Hill - ISBN 9781684113323 – The blue book - I'm not drawn like others to reading the bible; so much of it is left up to interpretation. It was Law Of Success that helped to clear my mind. Everything you need to navigate through the struggles of life is in there.   No agenda, no interpretations, just straight out lessons that should be taught in every high school across the country.

13 Valentines – Don Endriss – Ahhhhh, I saved the best for last.   This is how I thought a love story should be written. When people ask me about love, I tell them, "I wrote the book!" 13Valentines.com ISBN 13: 9780578010304

www.ingramcontent.com/pod-product-compliance
Lightning Source LLC
Chambersburg PA
CBHW020351290526
45785CB00005B/2224